Confessions of a Heroin Addict

Confessions of a Heroin Addict

Dr. Renee Denobrega, DNP, PMHNP

Copyright © 2019 by Dr. Renee Denobrega, DNP, PMHNP.

Library of Congress Control Number:		2019904800
ISBN:	Hardcover	978-1-7960-2911-6
	Softcover	978-1-7960-2910-9
	eBook	978-1-7960-2909-3

All rights reserved. No part of this book may be reproduced or transmitted in any form or by any means, electronic or mechanical, including photocopying, recording, or by any information storage and retrieval system, without permission in writing from the copyright owner.

The views expressed in this work are solely those of the author and do not necessarily reflect the views of the publisher, and the publisher hereby disclaims any responsibility for them.

Any people depicted in stock imagery provided by Getty Images are models, and such images are being used for illustrative purposes only.
Certain stock imagery © Getty Images.

Print information available on the last page.

Rev. date: 04/22/2019

To order additional copies of this book, contact:
Xlibris
1-888-795-4274
www.Xlibris.com
Orders@Xlibris.com
794421

CONTENTS

Preface vii

Chapter 1   The Neuro-pathophysiology of Addiction.....................1

Chapter 2   Genetics and Addiction 5

Chapter 3   Substance Abuse and Mood Disorders 7

Chapter 4   Mental Health Disorders 13

Chapter 5   Story Time..17

Chapter 6   Story Time 2...23

Chapter 7   Story Time 3...29

Chapter 8   Final Story and Conclusion...33

Conclusion and Final Remarks...37

PREFACE

Heroin is a preposterous offender to the health and prosperity of its users and subsequently, heroin has contributed to the influx of drug abusers. I do not desire to delve into statistics, epidemiological, or historical elements in terms of who, what, where, when and why, yet I will personify this substance and share my observations of its obvious criminal profile and the threat it poses to human existence.

Working as a medical and psychiatric provider in various substance rehabilitation facilities, I have managed to obtain first hand, or rather, a front row seat into the arena of the opioid epidemic. There seems to be a scientific paranormal and peculiar mechanism of action as to how heroin operates against its target population. Most of the victims are those who are weakened by childhood trauma, ancestral patterns of addiction, peer pressure, have little access to psychological care, physiological dependence, and lastly, a weakened will (i.e., the inability to say "no.") Oftentimes, it's not even a matter of saying no because it's gradually introduced, starting from alcohol to marijuana and to becoming socially acceptable in most of its affiliate settings.

In addition to the social dynamics, there is a synergistic effect of endogenous chemicals that tends to alleviate emotional distress instantaneously, and thereby individuals depend on this biological feedback for temporary pleasure, recreation, and its anti- depressive properties. A majority of heroin addicts have some form of unresolved or repressed emotional childhood trauma and faulty upbringing. On the other hand, they will acquire traumatic events during their active addiction and find themselves depending on the substance to provide temporary relief in the midst of psychological commotion that was subsequent to the use of this controlled substance.

Some patients, who have or had physical ailments, are prescribed oral preparations of opioids by a physician, but without regard for their social class, their addiction still becomes inevitable. Now, how do prescribed oral concentrations of opioids lead to IV heroin use? This will be discussed in the following chapter that will explain the physiology of addiction.

Another phenomenon is that prescribers may attempt to titrate the dose of the prescribed opioid, or they may abruptly stop the patient—if they are pending legal investigations against their practice. There are several doctors who've lost their license as a result of creating a moneymaking mill behind prescribing these opioids. These practitioners can have over one thousand compliant patients in their database. Keep in mind that these patients don't miss appointments; a health care consumer may miss their dentist or chiropractic appointment, but when they're being prescribed an addictive medication, it's like the hungry rat and cheese phenomenon that no matter what life events may occur, these patients will not miss their opioid appointment.

These type of practitioners intentionally prescribe medications that chemically puppeteer their patients in order to generate great revenues. This was an old strategy by physicians who have started their own practice, independent from hospital affiliations and have the desire to stay in business—so I was told. These doctors almost became manic in their prescriptive efforts to supposedly relieve the patient's pain. However, once these fraudulent practices are reprimanded, that leaves one thousand plus patients without addictive medication to treat their actual or somatic pain.

Remember that all people, regardless of their race and social status, can acquire addictions, and thereby, these physicians become addicted to making money and oftentimes, they lose sight of adhering to ethical standards of professional practice. Shortly after, these patients find a quick and easy way to avoid withdrawal from this substance. Hence, they end up purchasing these drugs from street pharmacists.

CHAPTER 1

The Neuro-pathophysiology of Addiction

There are compulsory and compensatory circuits or pathways in the brain. These pathways are highly indicative of dopaminergic action, and they are linked to the human's capability to experience pleasure. Any activity or exogenous chemical that is highly addictive will yield to compulsive and or impulsive behavioral expression. Usually, people want to be at peace or in a state of pleasure. No one typically wants to endure pain or stress, and no one wants to be uncomfortable, so anything that produces pleasure tend to be desired by human beings.

Compulsive to impulsive drug use followed by extreme addiction and tolerance involves the dysregulation of chemicals hanging out in the reward circuits. Just like any regulatory process or law, there should be an on and off button or a sensory mechanism similar to a thermostat. A negative feedback loop is another way to describe this systematic process—when one goes up, some regulator must circumvent in order to bring it down. Another common pathway in the brain is the reinforcement and reward segment, which is hypothesized to function like the mesolimbic pathway.

Other crucial pathways for reward and subsequent behaviors are the ventral tegmental area and the nucleus accumbens. These pathways are involved in regulating responses that consist of different types of emotional highs, such as the natural high after winning a race, marathon, or a profound academic achievement. There are also behaviorally induced highs, such as gambling, and a substance-induced high.

Drug abuse tends to release an exponential amount of dopamine in this mesolimbic pathway in comparison to a natural high. This type of high is linked to chronic behavioral adaptations and clinical manifestations such as cravings, dependence, preoccupation, and withdrawal syndromes. With perpetual use of the substance stimulated by compulsivity, the gratification eventually diminishes over time and yields a tolerance to the substance— meaning that the abuser will require a higher dose in order to feel the initial high. Usually, most patients who become chronic substance abusers will be psychologically and chemically programmed to pursue similar states of euphoria even during sobriety. For example, these patients who want to remain sober will usually have to be medicated with other psychopharmacological agents to induce particular chemical exchanges in order to achieve some mood-altering effect.

Also, I found that some patients who choose to abstain from substance abuse and trial sobriety tend to acquire some form of dependence on activities that would produce some kind of high. For example, they may work excessively, get into weight lifting or excessive shopping, or seek some type of involvement in stimulating activities as the drug proposed. IV heroin abuse has an overwhelming addictive profile due to its route of entry and expedition to the brain. Usually, the speed in which the drug crosses the brain barrier yields a stronger reinforcing effect. This is also due to the drug's onset of action followed by the stimulation of dopamine firing.

Dopamine is involved in naturally reinforcing and/or adapting behavior, such as eating, sleeping, drinking, defecating, itching, and even sneezing. My simple explanation for this is that the body needs to encourage you to do certain voluntary functions; otherwise, you won't do it. For example, defecation is important, and if there isn't some type of pleasure or relieving factor in performing this natural function, then people just won't do it. Therefore, the body would not be able to exist with voluntary cooperation.

Dopamine is highly indicative of encouraging the human being to perform certain tasks. There are different degrees of pleasure, and usually, we associate pleasure in risk taking or secretive naughty behaviors. However, pleasure is also a form of ease at its lowest potential. In so many words, there are degrees of pleasure. Some people will max out pleasure-inducing chemicals that are almost like a machine on overdrive, performing several different types of pleasurable behaviors and producing an overwhelming manufacture of chemicals and fluctuation of dopamine working on several aspects of the reward pathways of the brain.

For example, some people will take different combinations of drugs that work on different receptors in different parts of the brain, thereby triggering different releases of dopamine and other chemicals. Some people will have wild sex while doing drugs, eat pleasurable foods, attend parties, and engage in fun social activities, thereby overwhelming their system. These activities produce dysregulatory responses and will trigger increase in risk-taking behaviors as the brain's executive functioning is disabled. There are medications that can block or occupy these receptors from engaging such chemicals, and thereby, the recipient may not feel the euphoric potentials of the drug with these blocking agents. However, if patients are conditioned to being high depending on their social influences, then then may overturn their sobriety and easily overdose in an attempt to bypass the medication that was probably prescribed to assist in sustaining sobriety.

Drug seekers are not necessarily people who just wants to be a menace to society; usually, there are several factors involved in this inherent behavior. Other factors are genetics, temperaments, personality types, socioeconomics, childhood trauma, other forms of social and emotional trauma, psychological components, and other psychiatric or behavioral disorders.

CHAPTER 2

Genetics and Addiction

We have to remember that human physiology is a dynamic organism with millions, perhaps billions, of processes that simultaneously interfaces with complicated organ systems and regulatory functions. These functions are orchestrated by the brain's instruction and pre-manufactured protein structures, DNA, enzymes, chromosomes, and all other forms of coding that may dictate behaviors.

Some behaviors are acquired, while others are innate. It's like a probability factor, and if both of your parents possess a particular trait that stood out, then more than likely, there is an increased likelihood of genetic adaptation associated with that behavioral trait. This will be passed down to their children. So remember, the stronger the degree of a particular trait, the greater the probability that these genes will be expressed. For example, if both of your parents had a type A personality—they were determined, hardworking, tenacious, motivated, acquired a knack for reading, learning, and excelling in their perspective interests or subjects—then more than likely, their children will exhibit some or all of these qualities.

Now, let's tie this in to parents who were chronic drug and alcohol abusers. Drugs were their affiliation from childhood and straight on to adulthood—all of their life endeavors revolved around drugs or alcohol. Believe it or not, these clients do exist, and more than likely, their children will encounter alcoholism or drug addiction. It is estimated that the human genome contains about twenty to thirty thousand genes within three million base pairs of DNA on twenty-three chromosomes. The concern is not the quantity of genes that we have because obviously, there's so many peers and molecular configurations; instead, it's the genes that are activated and expressed. Genes are involved in every organ process, and patients acquire genetic disorders because there was an inherited glitch in a particular molecular mechanism, affecting neurotransmission and other structural components of cellular functions. This is just a snippet of an intelligible yet complex system in the human anatomy. Therefore, when we observe human behaviors, it's best to go beyond face value since your body is an intelligent organism that adapts to its environment on a molecular level.

All of these processes that are invisible to the human eye have intelligence. Human behaviors directly impact these intelligible microorganisms, and if there's a prolonged history of exposure to certain types of behaviors, then there is a greater degree of genetic expression that will be passed down to the next generation. Usually, when you go to the doctor for an initial physical examination, one of the first questions are about your family history. That's because if your parents developed cancer or any particular medical condition, you are at a higher risk for developing that same condition. Please keep in mind that when dealing with human beings, we all have a background. Some of us are not familiar with our family history —perhaps only one or two generations back— thereby, some of our behaviors are programmed, coded, or hardwired.

We are not dissimilar to computer systems. As a matter of fact, I would like to say that computer programs and software are probably a mimic of the human brain. Hopefully, if you're a clinician reading this text, you have a little more understanding and compassion for certain patients that you may encounter who have odd or peculiar behaviors that are frustrating or difficult to treat. More than likely, this person has adapted a certain condition within their upbringing, or it could be a chemical adaptation from inherited biological factor.

CHAPTER 3

Substance Abuse and Mood Disorders

From my experience in dealing with substance abuse disorders, it is more than likely that you are dealing with an individual who has been significantly traumatized. I'm talking about life-changing childhood trauma coupled with dysfunctional social dynamics. When a human being grows in such an unstable environment, there are several negative impacts that will affect normal physiological processes within their neurochemistry.

When a person's brain has been traumatized, there are several processes and segments of the brain that are injured, and this is where psychological disorders occur. In my practice, I have seen patients with posttraumatic stress disorder (PTSD) who have acquired vast expressions of mental health disturbances. Usually, they have seen a psychiatrist or a child therapist at some point, and they are more than likely diagnosed with ADD, oppositional defiance, or some form of mood dysregulation. After a trial of stimulants and mood-altering psychotropics, individuals with such a traumatic history will eventually find drugs. Oftentimes, I find patients in which the trauma has been compounded. I will get into case scenarios in the following chapters; however, after trying several psychiatric medications with lack of proper follow-up and lack of a stable family dynamics, the patient will be decompensated.

Marijuana is extremely addictive with a high degree of dependence, and probably 80% of the people I treat are concomitantly using marijuana. Marijuana is easily distributed and is readily available, so usually, individuals who have been traumatized will resort to this easily accessible drug or substances to modulate emotional or stressful responses. Once a person starts to use a substance that is mind-altering and works on dopamine in those rewards circuits in the brain, usually, it will open the door for them to try other substances that engage in those exact processes in particular circuitries to enhance the effect. Oftentimes, these mind-altering and addictive substances are sedative, and they can impair memory and cause a great deal of apathy or numbness. The reason substance abuse is highly attractive to a person who has a lot of unresolved trauma and stress is so they may not feel the intensity of those emotions and be able to suppress them with the alleged mood-altering properties.

The problem occurs when the abusers has to depend on that substance because it's usually short-lived. As soon as the substance is metabolized and excreted from the body, all of their symptoms return—if not worse. Oftentimes, children will have behavioral disturbances as a result of substance abuse, and parents are not aware. Even among adults, when treated by a psychiatrist or other psychiatric provider, their substance abuse, often times, is not disclosed. Patients may present a conglomerate of symptoms, and thereby the doctor will diagnose the patient with several condition, but more than likely, the root cause is a substance abuse.

This is why a good therapist is very important because it boils down to a savvy and rather astute provider to sit with a patient and pick apart behaviors followed by delving into the deep ocean of their childhood history. There are different degrees of trauma that impacts people in different ways, and some individuals are a little more resistant, and they have conformed to their trauma-filled environment. At some point, trauma becomes a norm, while for others traumatic distress will cause severe insecurities and fears and thereby impacts the patient's world view or self-esteem. This concept is psychologically damaging and another constituent to chronic substance abuse as it temporarily manages those fearful stimuli.

Another personality that I've noticed that particularly abuses alcohol are those with avoidant personality disorders and those with social anxiety. These individuals are extremely uncomfortable among groups and social settings. Engaging with others and building friendships are terrifying for them. They are usually uncomfortable with themselves, and perhaps they were programmed at some point during childhood with experiences that gave them a faulty sense of self. People who suffer with extreme social phobias and discomfort in social settings tend to misuse alcohol to mellow them out, and thereby, an addiction is more than likely going to follow.

Oftentimes, any substance that unnaturally manipulates dopamine will have mood-altering effects. When a person becomes addicted, their main motivation is to procure more drugs. Addiction also involves an unbalanced and dysfunctional spikes in dopamine. Dopamine is involved in motivation, anticipation of a reward, preoccupation, obsession, and overstimulation. These behaviors will develop into impulsivity and compulsive drug use. When these behaviors continue to escalate—usually as a result of high doses of a particular stimulant—a person will become restless, irritable, hyperactive, and begin to panic. At higher doses of particular stimulants, there is a greater likelihood to experience hypertension, increase in heart rate, hyperthermia, and/or respiratory depression. As doses increase, abusers exhibit manic behaviors, and when doses begin to decrease, the patient will begin to withdraw and become extremely irritable and depressed. Some individuals may experience suicidality, irrationality, and erratic psychotic manifestations. The depression also kicks in after the individual have spent all their money and performed shameful task in order to obtain the income for this drug—it's like reality kicks in. As I mentioned earlier, your main focus, motivation, and drive is to obtain that drug; thereby, your executive, administrative, and/or higher functioning processes of brain are temporarily shut down.

During an addiction, there's no reciprocity of emotions, and there's no give-and-take. There's no "if I do this, I'm going to hurt that."

Usually, when a person is in an active addiction, they will go at all costs to obtain that drug. They will do things outside of their character, outside of their social norm, and outside of their religious belief systems. They are obsessed with the drug and the mechanical manipulation of a powerful agnostic effect. These chemicals acting in a particular pathway of the brain is on overdrive. Usually, when these behaviors are exhibited, they will be classified under a drug-induced bipolar disorder. As their body gets used to the chemicals in the behaviors associated with the illicit use of these chemicals, then even with sobriety, a person may exhibit some of these behaviors because now, they are acquired. This is why psychotherapy coupled with psychotropic medications are important to reprogram the brain after a person has chronically abused substances. Some of the psychological dysfunctions will impact their ability to sleep as it is disturbs circadian rhythms, and the person will usually have to take another substance to put them to sleep, and whatever that substance is, it's usually psychoactive and habit-forming that the person becomes addicted to another substance to treat another symptom caused by another illicit substance.

It's very important for doctors to screen for substance abuse when a patient postulates a series of symptoms or syndromes. An organic bipolar disorder should not have any substance abuse factored in to their symptoms. Bipolar mania is a series of symptoms over a period of time, usually hyperactivity, a surge of motivation, grandiosity, hypersexuality, excessive behavior such as shopping and cleaning, insomnia, and an inflated sense of self. This mania will catapult into delusional thinking and psychosis where the person begins to lose touch with reality, and they can also develop hallucinations. There are theories that during mania and psychosis associated with schizophrenia, dopamine is increased in certain regions of the brain, and this is why most antipsychotics will block dopamine by shutting down the schizophrenic symptoms.

This is why it's important to have a good therapist and a doctor who will accurately diagnose your disorders and determine whether it's coming from a substance or from an organically inherited disorder. If a person has organic bipolar disorder, there are theories that a regular antidepressant can induce mania or anger, and thereby this individual should be on mood stabilizer as monotherapy. Usually, a person with a substance abuse disorder who has acquired a bipolar disease will be able to function with an antidepressant and a mood stabilizer. Remember that every individual has their own goals or personal beliefs in regard to their psychiatric care as it relates to their substance abuse disorder. Some patients will tell me that they don't want any medications at all, and 90% of them actually need something to assist with maintaining sobriety because depression usually follows the cessation of a substance. If these individuals use substance abuse to suppress anger from some major traumatic past, then during periods of sobriety, all of those emotions will resurrect. Usually, when a person is acquiring some periods of sobriety, their life is in shambles—they've lost their apartment, their job, their marriage, their children, their stability, and so on and so forth. This can be extremely depressing; hence, when treating substance abuse disorders followed by sobriety, it is very important to encourage the individual to embrace a holistic approach. Oftentimes, they will need to adjust their diet, they will need to engage in psychotherapy, they will need to ensure that there's a good connection between their history, their personality, and the therapist, otherwise the person will not feel comfortable enough to disclose details in regards to their life and their history, and it would defeat the purpose of therapy.

Family support is necessary. However, 50% of individuals who have substance abuse disorders have exhausted their families' resources and patience. I often recommend patients in this situation to find a church or support group who are family-oriented so that this individual can develop family bonds and ties with other individuals who are not relatives.

Finding faith is a highly suggested in those who seek recovery. It's obvious that there are spiritual and supernatural forces involved in human affairs and the course of our history. Submitting to one's faith in God brings about a dependence on a higher power that can help them receive a certain degree of healing as they begin the process in conforming to a belief in a God that loves them regardless.

This element of recovery can be highly satisfying to the addict as oftentimes, they feel alone and ashamed of the poor choices that they've made. The ministry of Christ highlights the concept of forgiveness and restoration. During the lowest parts of a person's life, they will need to be reminded that all human beings, regardless of their imperfections or choices have done wrong. There are several factors e.g., environmental factors, genetic factors, and others that will offer substance abuse as an option for "self-therapy. So before a person casts a stone, they have to remember that we are not without sin.

CHAPTER 4

Mental Health Disorders

Opioid addicts are no stranger to trauma and mental health disorders. About 90 percent of the cases of people abusing highly addictive chemicals such as heroin will result in them having a psychiatric disorder. IV substance abuse is extraordinarily addictive because of its explosive influx of dopamine in particular and other chemicals. It crosses over the brain barriers faster and does not need to be absorbed through the stomach and into the intestines, the liver, and other processes that distributes the blood throughout the system. Hence, it hits the brain faster, and it has a ceiling affect where it skyrockets to certain receptors that are involved in the neurotransmission of the high. This high usually doesn't last as long, and thereby, dealers tend to add other chemicals to reproduce other types of high in addition to the heroin and opioid high. Remember, drug dealers and their entourage or enterprise would like to sustain their business, and they usually try to get drugs that people will like and thus continue to use them as their primary drug supplier.

Depression is a series of negative symptoms. People can have major depression, mild, moderate, and severe, with periods of remission and episodic breaks. Depression starts to escalate when a person is not able to function normally, if they are unable to find hope then suicidality is up for consideration. As depression transitions from mild to moderate then an abuser will often times seek help. If the antidepressants fail, then depression tends to persist more often.

People who take drugs and have substance abuse disorders and are prescribed antidepressants at the same time can be very dangerous. They will go to their therapist or psychiatrist and claim that the medications are working yet fail to disclose their substance abuse or dependence in drugs.

Depression usually involves a series of symptoms: excessive sleeping, fatigability, lack of motivation, lack of hope, lack of joy, despair, depressed mood, isolation, loneliness, decreased sunlight exposure, and discontinuation of their passion or the usual activities that brings joy to them. One can become distant and despondent from family members, and one can also experience a decreased sex drive or interest with their partner. There are also the involvement of self-esteem issues and excessive guilt and shame. When a person is being diagnosed with depression, the doctor should make sure that there are no other underlying physiological causes, such as thyroid disease and vitamin D deficiency, anemia, Parkinson's disease, and other physical complaints. Furthermore, fibromyalgia and/or a history of gastric bypass surgery have been linked to depression, and thus, a doctor should check those levels to ensure that a person is not depressed because of some deficiency that simply needs adjusted order to reroute depression.

Women undergoing menopause and/or have hormonal changes as a result of a hysterectomy are other known causes of depression. Other atypical forms of depression can be found in someone that exhibits poorly controlled anger or automatic negative thought patterns. Depression can be the underlying reason why some people tend to be angry and complain all of the time. They seem to be unkind and lacking in love and affection. They can be prideful in some respects, or their negative emotional expressions. Oftentimes, people don't want to admit it that they're depressed and can be offended by it. They tend to avoid the topic, and hence, treatment will be delayed. In order to circumvent the cycle and or get wind of depression, one must be open to acknowledge these symptoms.

There is another disorder that was once called dysthymia, but now, it's a persistent depressive disorder. The person having this disorder does not have episodic depressive episodes. They exhibit about 50% of the major depressive symptoms, and they're able to function normally, but usually, they experience constant (perhaps for a time greater than two years) low mood, apathy, or lack of interest in things that they normally like to do (if there are any). Remember that these disorders can be genetically inclined.

Anxiety tends to manifest independent of depression. However, if a person's anxiety is poorly controlled or if insomnia is poorly controlled, then it could lead to depression and severe mental illness. Oftentimes, when individuals have not sought psychiatric help, they tend to use alcohol or street drugs that are readily available to cope with their symptoms. Anxiety can stem from unresolved situations or repressed trauma and fear.

People with anxiety disorders tend to worry a lot, and they create a pathway in the brain that is specific to worrying. Worrying can have varying degrees, such as worrying about what you're going to wear tomorrow or worrying about major problems like how you are going to pay your bills after recently losing a job. Usually, the nervous system is stimulated, and a person with anxiety tends to either have a constant or fluctuating state of restlessness and autonomic hyperactivity that can trigger heart palpitations, upset stomach, racing thoughts, agitation, and easily overwhelmed and loss of mental control.

Insomnia tends to have an underlying effect on mood and anxiety. Sometimes, repressed fears or concerns may not be in the forefront of your thought processes, but there are quite a few unresolved situations and another dimension of your existence that tend to harbor all of the weight or heaviness that you are feeling.

Some people have sleep-wake cycle disturbances where their schedules are off or perhaps when they shift schedules at work. Others are on medications that affect their nervous system, and the schedule or timing in which they take their medication needs to be adjusted in order to reduce their anxiety and thereby induce sleep.

Opioids will cause insomnia. They can help with sleep, but when you're no longer able to continue to take a particular dose of the opioid, it can cause hypersomnia. Another common cause of insomnia is excessive snoring and or obstructive sleep apnea. Oftentimes, patients are aware of the fact that they snore at night, and they're simply not able to breathe during certain periods of their sleep phase. This alerts other processes in the brain to wake that person up so that they can catch their breath.

Other causes of insomnia are night terrors. Some people have trauma that they really live particularly at night. Thus, psychotherapy is important so that the person can process these traumatic events through higher executive systems within the brain and thus stimulate rationality and understanding so that the repressed traumas are not relived particularly at night, causing someone insomnia.

CHAPTER 5

Story Time

During my interviews with patients and extensive and brief psychiatric evaluations, I have heard some of the most outrageous stories. I will advise all mental health therapist to process their trauma accordingly because oftentimes, the experiences that patients share will trigger some of your personal distress, and you can decompensate quickly.

The first scenario I'd like to discuss is a time when a patient came to me and proposed this question, "Why should I live? My mother was a crackhead. She prostituted at me at the age of five to her homosexual friends who were also cocaine abuse. I contracted HIV as a result of my mother's ridiculous and psychotic obsession during her active cocaine addiction. Now, I am a substance abuser and I am depressed. I am reliving trauma. What should I do?"

I had another patient who shared an equally tragic situation in which his mother was a psychotic alcohol abuser. Oftentimes, patients look at alcohol as being the least life-altering drug, but alcohol can mimic the exact behavior induced by other drugs. It can be worse than heroin addiction because alcohol is a gatekeeper, and oftentimes, people will initiate their abuse history with alcohol or marijuana. Once they're intoxicated, then their defenses are low, and they're open to trying other types of drugs. Anyways, this patient told me that his mother had him perform oral sex on her since the age of three. When I heard this story,

I think the earth stopped moving. I asked him, "Can you explain to me what you just said?" He said around the age of three or four or five, when he was drinking his bottle, all he knew is that his face would be in a particular position, and he was just encouraged to lick. This type of sexual abuse occurred until the age of twelve. His brother was also coerced into having sexual relationships with his mother.

Usually, when this type of abuse takes place, the victim will acquire sexual confusion and identity disorders, and they will have poor sexual impulse control and often engage in sexual activities with others at an early age. At some point during their childhood upbringing, they were not able to process the awkwardness in the criminality of perversion because they were introduced to this activity by their own mother. Sometimes, these patients are not aware that what they're doing is wrong. However, there is and intensity in the regulation of their moods and emotions because on some dimension of their psyche, they know that something isn't right. Needless to say, this patient acquired an opioid and a cocaine addiction. He was one of my most profound patients. After making telling me his story, he said, "I forgive my mother because I've realized that something terribly disastrous and equally disturbing trauma must've taken place in her life in which she perpetrated." How would you respond to this?

Another patient, in which the story took an interesting turn for the worse, was sexually abused at the age of fifteen. His father was schizophrenic, and he attempted suicide by hanging on more than one occasion. This followed his repeated traumatic upbringing. After one of his suicide attempts he reported having a near-death experience in which he saw his grandparents who have passed on and told him that it was not his time.

After he came out of the closet and was" resurrected from the dead," his father said, "I knew you were in there. I was just waiting for you to die so I can call the ambulance." Another event was when he found out that his child hood molester was applying for a job at the local grocery store in which he was employed. He informed the managers about what that potential employee had done. However, they all made a laughing stock out of him.

Needless to say, he acquired a substance abuse disorder, as well as inappropriate subsequent behaviors. As he spoke to the nurses at the rehab, he was finally able to cry, and he shared his interest in music which became his escape. Prior to the rehab, he had a suicide attempt, yet he denied it to us and claimed that he will not hurt himself. Apparently, he was having of social issues at the rehab as he was the only black or mixed race person there at the time, and some made racial comments that were inappropriate. He was ticking some people off, and his girlfriend who he cheated on was Caucasian, and her family was not in agreement with their relationship, was not supportive of his rehabilitation, and had a hard time forgiving him for the infidelity or his disloyalty. She went against her family's beliefs and views, yet he ended up breaking her heart. He did not have an explanation as to why he cheated; he really loved this girl.

He opened up to me about certain things. However, I was new to working in the substance abuse arena at that time, and I was warned that we had to make sure that we kept our boundaries between patients; otherwise, I could lose my job. I tried to talk to him about faith and giving his life to God. He shared some spiritual experiences in church in which the worship and manifestation of God's glory was immensely and extremely phenomenal. He felt it throughout his body, yet he was not able to continue his walk with God.

I will never forget the Jesus tattoo and the scripture on his forearm. I gave him some reading material, and I tried to encourage him to pursue his musical dreams. I remember him telling me that he didn't want to go back to jail because he had been incarcerated quite a few times, and that was also another magnetic force that he couldn't seem to escape. I told him that I would pray for him to never go back to jail. Well, I got a call that night, and in so many words, my prayers did come to pass. He did never go back to jail; instead, he hung himself in the rehab. They rushed him to the hospital, and he was in life-support.

I was extremely distressed. I spoke to my children at home about the situation, and we just continued to pray and hoped that he would come out of the coma. I had several dreams and visionary and counters that night which gave me some insight into what actually took place.

One day, my son told me, "Mom, do you remember that boy who hung himself on a tree? He told me to tell you that he's OK and he said hi." I asked my son what he looked like, and he said, "He looks like our dad." His dad has soft and curly thick hair, and that patient did as well. When I called the hospital, I found that he did expire.

I've had another patient who shared an equally disturbing story. He had a few years of sobriety, under his belt and was rehabilitating from his murder-filled upbringing in Puerto Rico. His son was recently murdered, and it triggered all of his dysfunctional, unresolved emotions, and tragic upbringing. He shared with me that his initial response was to go and kill the person who killed his son, but instead, he relapsed on drugs and admitted himself to rehab.

He talked about growing up in the projects in Puerto Rico. He was forced to chop up bodies, ears, eyes, and noses. He may have been gang affiliated, as he mentioned to me that the perpetrators of these criminal activities forced him into disposing the bodies in such a manner or else they would kill him. I believe he was also connected to a drug cartel, and he said in his country, in the low socioeconomic regions, death was imminent, and there would be at least six dead bodies every day. One time, as he was cutting up a dead body of a woman (who I guess ratted out a drug dealer or spilled some information that she should not have and the consequence was death, as he was chopping up her body), he heard her spirit saying, "Why? Why me? Why am I like this?" This patient had also served a significant amount of time in jail, and he had witnessed multiple traumatic situations. What do you say to a patient like this? How would you come for the human beings coming from this type of a background?

Another patient I had from Puerto Rico also grew up in the projects and had served a significant amount of jail time in his country. I was told that a person can be sentenced to prison from ninety days to sixteen years in Puerto Rico, if I'm not mistaken. That was that very patient the criminal activity that takes place in jail in their system continues to for them more time, and there is no escape from crime in the present system. He said he could never sleep, and had to constantly watch his back. To him, humans were like monsters, and junkies who retaliated with pride and superiority gain drug-related competition. After witnessing several murders, he acquired schizophrenia. He described that the voice would interrupt his conversation with others, and when he tried to avoid listening to this hallucinatory voice, it would give him an excruciating headache. The voice once told him, "I'm not gonna stop until you kill yourself."

Oftentimes, he personified this voice because it was almost as if it was another entity that lives inside of him. Once the voice took over, he would be under the influence of anger and other intense emotions, and he would have no recollection of what took place afterwards. Obviously, substance abuse didn't help this patient. He was heavily medicated and was on psychiatric medications, but he feared this entity would take over and that he would kill his family and then himself. He was married and loved his wife and family very much, but he could not understand what had possessed him. Needless to say, he acquired an opioid and cocaine addiction. What would you say to a patient with this kind of complaint? As a human being with compassion and love, how would you comfort someone undergoing this strange form of suffering?

CHAPTER 6

Story Time 2

Another story was of a young man who was repeatedly raped by his uncle. His uncle was had a sexual intercourse with him at a very young age, and it went on nonstop for years. I asked the patient, "Well, why didn't you tell anyone?" He replied, "Oftentimes, people would not believe me, or I did tell them and nothing happened."

This individual became homosexual, and he became an escort and a prostitute. He talked about the strange fetishes that some of his clients possessed. One of his clients requested for him to defecate on his face, and he would have them go to the store and or at McDonald's to eat a lot of food, then he will give him laxatives so that he can have a bowel movement on his face. This patient received thousands of dollars for this. He witnessed the man wipe his face with his bowel contents and receive an erection followed by an orgasm.

Another client of his would request high amounts of cocaine prior to sexual activity. The patient mentioned to me that one of his clients was highly competitive, and he was forced to be flexible in order to support her lifestyle. This particular client lavished him with thousands of dollars a month, furnished his apartment, and the like. Some of his clients were attorneys, lawyers, doctors, and other high profile individuals. After he was highly intoxicated with cocaine, his client would have him make a fist and penetrate his anus in a particular way that would give him an orgasm. Another one of his clients requested for him to find another prostitute "who was homosexual and HIV positive." They had to bring the results of their HIV test so that he could have sex with them. This person apparently had a family and children, but this was one of those strange fetishes.

Needless to say, this patient required a cocaine and opioid addiction. He was also bipolar with chronic PTSD and needed to be heavily medicated during his periods of sobriety.

During the course of an addiction, trauma is usually compounded, so a person most likely already have a significant childhood trauma. I've heard so many malaise stories from patients who were prostituted by their parents for drugs, patients who were part of sex trafficking rings as a child, patients who were brutally abused by their parents, and individuals who conceive children from their parents. In addition to that degree of despicable and unbelievable trauma, during their addiction, they've lost many friends and loved ones because of substance abuse.

I've heard many stories of individuals who lost their loved ones, their fiancés, and their spouses. As a result, they sometimes are found hanging in the basement or with an overdose of drugs. One profound story that stood out to me was a man who was about to perform oral sex to his girlfriend. She had a cardiac condition, and they were abusing cocaine and other stimulants as he was performing oral sex. She said, "Wait a minute," and then went into a deep silence followed by intense snoring. I'm assuming that he didn't think anything of it because when you're abusing opioids and benzodiazepines, you can doze off and alternate between alertness to drowsiness and sedation to a deep snore. Needless to say, she never woke back up again. Some of my questions were, "What do you tell the police? Will you tell their family?"

I've had patients who were disowned by their partner's family because their partner's family looked at them as the perpetrator since they were the last person who saw their partners alive. Also, they did drugs with their partner who died, so they have to live with that guilt and shame. Oftentimes, the opioids would give them a degree of apathy, and they can talk to me about those situations with a straight face.

I had two patients in this situation in which they were hunting, and the gun had a little glitch as they were messing around with it. One patient of mine blew the head off of his best friend. The patient performed CPR, called the cops, and tried to revive him in whatever way he could, but his best wasn't good enough. Needless to say, he acquired an opioid addiction. What do you say to a patient like that? How do you come for a human being with that degree of distress?

I have another story of a patient who also had to perform sexual acts. His mother also made him addicted to drugs, and she prostituted him as a child. She taught him how to shoot her up with IV opioids. One day, he shot it up, and she never woke back up again. I asked him, "Did you do that intentionally?" He said, "I don't know," followed by a, "No comment."

He was disowned and persecuted by all of his family members because they accused him of killing his mother by not administering the safe amount of opioids. However, no one thought about the fact that she was prostituting him and was making him perform oral sex on her. He should not have been administering IV drugs to her in the first place, so why should he be responsible for her death? Needless to say, this patient acquired an opioid addiction with an unstable lifestyle and was homeless and without a comfortable place or family to love him. What do you tell a patient like that? How do you advise them, and how do you come for them?

Readers, if you are a therapist or someone considering to study this field, you might want to learn different therapeutic modalities that are not in textbooks because you don't want to be robotic in your approach in assisting the recovery of patients with PTSD. I would offer spirituality as an element to the treatment since every human being possesses a soul and a spirit, and sometimes, encouraging their faith if they believe in God. Tell them the love of God that can renew and transform their lives. Offer supernatural aspects of healing from a generational cycle of negativity as a result of parents and grandparents who made poor choices and passed them on like curses. If a patient has faith, this would definitely be the time to stimulate their faith and not to take it away from them as oftentimes, all they have is their faith and it can save them. I've seen medications that mechanically alters the brain chemistry, and patients end up like zombies they are not able to feel anything, and even their movements are robotic and are chemically institutionalized.

High doses of certain psychiatric medications can take away the humanity of an individual, especially if it's not coupled with adequate psychotherapy. Oftentimes, I've met students entering the field of psychology because they have some psychiatric disorder or concerns of their own, and they enter into that field thinking that they'll heal on their own. Although this organized emotional process can perhaps help another person, I do not recommend going into this field for that reason. I would work instead on achieving some level of healing as I don't believe that a broken person who has repressed trauma can do well in delving into a field with people who may have suffered enormous tragedy and odd defying events.

When drug addicts get raped, tortured, and assaulted, the legal system usually dismisses it as they were probably going to engage in that activity anyway to get the drug. I had one patient who was raped by an Uber driver at the time when Uber had just first come out as a service a few years ago in the United States. Thus, she did not pursue any legal charges because she was a drug addict.

Another patient of mine was a young and beautiful Jewish girl. However, at a very young age, she was raped and sexually molested, and it went on for years. You kind of wonder how people survive that kind of torture from the ages of six to twelve. Oftentimes, family members patches things up and don't want to tell anyone. As a result, she acquired PTSD and schizophrenia.

She talked about the cats that are a part of her delusions, and a particular man and one of the cats in both her hallucinations and reality died recently. She did mention that at the rehab, she discussed some of the things that she saw in the unseen realm. She mentioned seeing a family outside the waiting room as if they were confused, and she also remembered seeing a child in the forest. Moreover, she talked about seeing a man hanging in the gym at the rehab. Apparently, this rehab was a treatment center years ago for tuberculosis, and some of the people she was seeing were obviously confused or still acting as a patient.

She tried to pursue legal accusations and prosecutions against her perpetrator, but her family was against it because of the fact that it was a family member who perpetrated this evil against her. She suffered with PTSD, schizophrenia, and a substance abuse disorder, and had she not indulged in that degree of malaise, she might've had a normal life. I told her that I could see her being a lawyer as she was an intelligent and a bright girl, yet her destiny was taken from her. How do you counsel a patient like this? What advice from a human being with compassion and care would you offer to a person with such a traumatic history?

I've heard horrible stories about how people dealing with the death of their children led them to an addiction to ease the pain. One patient told me that perhaps his three-year-old daughter was lying in her bed; however, she had like a canopy net above her bed in which all of her teddy bears were temporarily stored. Somehow, her head got caught into that canopy net, and he walked in on his three-year-old, already hanging dead. I believe this patient did have an addiction prior, and his wife also had an addiction. This compounded his addiction, and if he was already using drugs before, then after the incident, he was bound to use more.

Another tragedy I heard of was from a patient who mentioned how a driver had a heart attack and his car slid over into the sidewalk where my patient's daughter was riding her little bike, and this led to her demise. This patient acquired a substance abuse disorder, needless to say.

I've heard of another interesting story of a patient who was chronic alcoholic, and in the midst of intoxication, he was haphazardly near a machine of some sort that chopped off his legs. When he came to his senses, he found a new body. He shared with me that as part of the process to sobriety, he needed adequate psychiatric medications at an effective dose because he mentioned, "You know when you can't walk up the stairs? It gets discouraging after a while, and it can trigger depression, and perhaps that was the reason that prolonged my alcohol addiction."

CHAPTER 7

Story Time 3

I've heard a lot about traumatic experiences in prison. One of my patients shared a story with me about a prolonged prison sentence taking over a decade. I didn't delve into the details of his particular client, but it seemed to me like his prison sentence was a life-changing experience.

He was a very tall African-American man, and initially, I was afraid of him because of his height and the fact that he was a substance abuser. There weren't any panic buttons in the room. And if any of these patients got upset, then I could have gotten injured. Needless to say, he was probably one of the sweetest patients I've had thus far. He shared with me that sometimes in the prison, guards are the worst criminals. There was an inmate who was taken by the guards, and they housed him in a cell with three other men who were extremely dangerous. The size of the cell was probably of a medium to a small bathroom. Anyways, they sealed the door shut for three days. They killed that inmate and they all took turns sodomizing his body for about two days before they opened the door. My patient said that he was quiet in the hall witnessing this the whole time. Obviously, this patient acquired an opioid addiction and a cocaine addiction. What therapeutic strategy will you used to assist in the healing process of this patient?

I've had a few patients who shared some of their military trauma. One patient in particular went to the military and got quickly accelerated in his ranking because he was apparently a really good shooter. He recalled having to kill a ten-year-old because that ten-year-old child was more than likely loaded with weapons and/or explosives that were going to threaten the US troopers. I believe he may have mentioned something along the lines of the disturbance that he caused that family. Anyhow, shortly after, he got a phone call that his high school sweetheart and his ten-year-old daughter was killed in a motor vehicle accident. After that, he went savage, and he would kill every opponent that walked during the war. I believe he was medically discharged and obviously diagnosed with double PTSD. I managed to stabilize him because for some strange reason as I was in the middle of my session with him, I felt the presence of his wife who had passed on, and I shared with him some of the things I was feeling. It happened to bring some healing to his soul.

He was once a strong man of faith, and I encouraged him to reunite with his shared faith with his wife who had passed on with Christ. This provided a tremendous healing for him in addition to the medications that I prescribed him. I have not heard from him since then, but I know that prior to him coming into the room with me, he was suicidal, but he left smiling. I'm sure there were other things I said to him that I can't quite disclose nor do I remember, but my question to you, reader, is how would you respond if you are considering to enter into this field? What therapeutic options would you explore with a patient coming from that unique degree of trauma?

The worst-case scenario for me was about molestation and how the patients will disclose the details, such as a patient's uncle who used his penis as a hotdog and had the patient put, I believe, ketchup on it and created a little playful scenario. That patient also required an opioid addiction. I've also learned about a lot of families where incest is prevalent, and I've met some patients who were five years old when they were taught by their brother's girlfriend to perform oral sex on them.

I encourage you all to pay attention to children's behaviors because not all the times when a child is "acting out," it's simply ADHD. Sometimes, children are covering up sexual abuse. You have to be in tune with your client and build a therapeutic relationship in which trust is established, and through this, you will get to know them well enough that you won't be pointing fingers everywhere and accusing the wrong person(s). This is usually a major cause for substance abuse. As the child grows up, they soon realize that these sexual exploitations were extreme. Beware of childcare providers in childcare settings because sometimes, people take on these jobs for their strange interest in sexual relationships with children. They may not touch a child to date, but they may fantasize about it, so you want to be intuitive and not take things at face value. Some babysitters I was told were the perfect match, yet all along, they were perpetrators. Individuals who were molested often have gender identity issues or sexual confusion and/or active sexual stimulation with promiscuous behaviors.

Family members need to be mindful of other family members because sometimes, the perpetrators are the people you least expect. Sometimes, the perpetrators are other children. I've seen children being molested by other their peers, and sometimes it's their own sibling. I've heard stories of sibling harassments, where out of jealousy and envy, he feels strange emotions leading to sexual abuse. Oftentimes, parents do not want to deal with this. It's so tragic and mind blowing how they go into an immediate state of denial or shock because usually, there's no one to turn to. I do recommend getting into immediate therapy counseling. If you do not have a good rapport with your counselor or therapist, then immediately look for another one.

People who have been victims of sexual abuse often become abusers. I once had a patient tell me, "I have nieces and nephews, and anytime they go in the bathroom or play alone, I try not to find myself in the same space with them. I respect their privacy and not necessarily because I think that I would harm a child, but I just want to be cautious considering my history."

I've also noticed a strange phenomenon where at some point, the child receives pleasurable stimulation and engagement with the sexual activity from their perpetrator. They get confused as to why they're getting some pleasure out of it, and as they enter into adulthood, there experience intense guilt and shame. Oftentimes, I will have to explain to the patient that there were chemicals that were stimulated and other dynamic processes that take place in sexual activities and were thus manipulated to do certain aspects of sexual pleasure. Usually, the abuser would coerce them into sexual acts in which they will try to solicit and reciprocate pleasure. As a result, the child will respond biologically, and depending on the environment or the atmosphere that is created by the perpetrator, they can engage the child and program or teach them to cooperate. These are important key elements to be mindful of when you are working with children, caring for children, or have children. Likewise, if an adult who has experience with substance abuse or has a traumatic past discloses this type of information, giving you some background knowledge in terms of how the victims and the perpetrators behave, then you can explain this to the victim, and this will provide tremendous healing to their psyche and assist in their emotional control and regulation.

I often encourage my patients who discloses this degree of trauma by projecting a new positive future for them and offering ways on how they could turn this situation around and help other people. I do encourage self-healing first, and once again, I would not recommend a person to study psychology and attempt to become a full fledge independent therapist if there are a background of chronic sexual abuse and other forms of drama that they have yet to deal with.

Some therapists think that they'll be able to heal through their studies and help other people, but you have to help yourself first before helping other people. I'm sure that there are ways we can help people to some magnitude while we're still broken, but you will not be able to provide the best care for your client if you're not able to address some of your unresolved issues. As a matter of fact, it will trigger depression, anger, and other psychological distress. Some therapists end up relapsing if they have a substance abuse background as a result of some of their clients that they have to deal with.

CHAPTER 8

Final Story and Conclusion

There was a patient suffering with major depression. During her rehabilitation, she isolated herself. She didn't appear to have much social skills, and she had a history of eating disorder, chronic low self-esteem, and appeared to be a loner.

Upon initial examination, I noticed that she refused to look at me. Her eyes were fixed to the ceiling, and I figured that perhaps she was a little shy. I needed a little bit more time to establish a therapeutic environment in which there is some degree of trust and comfort between us. Mind you, I don't usually have much time to establish this type of a trusting environment. I will probably see them for about fifteen to twenty minutes; therefore, I must be sharp. I usually call it "emergency surgery" as I'm not there to build a long-term relationship with a patient; I'm there to diagnose, treat, and provide an immediate therapy.

Most patients in rehabs are there for about twenty-one to twenty-eight days, so you'll only see them one time. It's similar to going to the ER for an emergency procedure; you may never see that doctor again, and that doctor is not there to build a long-time rapport with you and is just there to immediately patch up the bleeding artery. Then they get sent to the next apartment to perform their task, which usually reinforces some degree of healing.

As the visit continued, I realized that ten to fifteen minutes later, this woman's eyes are still fixed to the ceiling, and I started to get offended. I thought to myself maybe there's something wrong with me. Her eyes were in a position where you could barely see the colored portion, and all you'd see was the white segment, and it was fixed to the ceiling. My second thought was maybe there's some intellectual disability or mental retardation and or perhaps some form of deformity that became apparent after a while.

She didn't answer all of my questions intelligently, although she had a fair insight and intellectual capacity. Finally, I just got a bold and asked her why she was not looking at me. Her response was, "I can't." That was a rather odd response, so I delved into why, and she mentioned that she hadn't looked at a human being since about the age of eighteen, and she was now about twenty-seven. There was some obvious childhood trauma that was reinforced when she gazed into the person's eyes, and her way of coping was to look up at the ceiling. Hence, the anatomy of her eyes adjusted to that position, and she was no longer able to voluntarily control her eye movements. After spending a little extra time with her, she got a little comfortable with me, and I asked her, "Can you try looking at me?" She tried, but she did not have the voluntary capacity to communicate to those nerves and muscles to focus in on looking directly at me.

I was told that she had a beautiful voice, with the most elaborate sounds of worship. This was her form of emotional breakthrough, but you can see that there was some darkness stemming from her background.

I was trying to suck every ounce of joy and happiness out of this woman. It was a follow-up visit, so I wasn't able to delve into the details of her history, nor was she forthcoming, so all I was able to do was take an educated guess in regard to the rhythm to her reason. I pose the question to you, readers: how would you approach this case?

Due to my lack of adequate time to spend with an individual that I will more than likely never see again, I tried to express professional love and care. I gave her I contact, I've validated her response, and I expressed joy and happiness in meeting a person like her. I empowered her gifts and her positive attributes to life and encouraged her to proceed in utilizing her whatever strengths she had that we were able to identify during that brief visit.

Another tip when counseling individuals going through deep emotional despair and anguish is knowing your boundaries. Sometimes, you want to take them into your home and shower them with love and affection—things that they have perhaps never had. However, once you're in a professional position, there are standards that you must abide to. Not all patients are going to be honest; some of them will absorb all of the shared sympathy within that short visit and in turn become manipulative. My visit may have been the only time in which they've experienced a little touch of hope.

On the other hand, I call this phenomenon that I'm about to mention the "underground railroad." There are some individuals you will encounter that will require you to go above and beyond the call of duty. There are many places in the world where policies and laws or regulations are implemented that hinders a person's freedom to choose. If missionaries were told that they must leave the country or else they will die, then there will be no more missionaries, and at that point, there's a choice that one has to make. Am I willing to sacrifice my life, my stability or my comfort for the sake of helping someone in need?

If Harriet Tubman did not pursue her route to freedom although it was illegal at that time, then her people would've been in bondage far longer than expected. Daniel was placed in the lion's den because an evil voice, under the influence of jealousy and envy, proposed a law to the king for the sole purpose of deterring Daniel from serving his God.

A therapeutic professional at some point must determine to what extent are they willing to go beyond professional boundaries—if at all necessary—in order to help another fellow human being. I would recommend acquiring wisdom and discernment. It takes experience to judge and determine whether an individual is safe for a therapeutic personnel to take any mild risk for the sake helping them.

Of course, as per the textbook, there should be *no* risks taken. However, we are in the real world where things are not cut and dry. You may encounter a patient who has many parallels to your life or an area of interest. Therefore, let's face it—the temptation to perhaps cross professional boundaries are real. You can never say that it will not happen, but once again, I will posit that as a therapeutic professional, you must use good judgment and try to remain as professional as possible.

CONCLUSION AND FINAL REMARKS

Substance abuse is a disorder that stems from any chemical that stimulates or agonizes the release of variable amounts of dopamine in particular pathways in the brain. These pathways are responsible for reward, compensation, and other reinforcing behaviors. The brain has its natural ability to regulate these chemicals. Usually, there are naturally rewarding behaviors that will increase levels of dopamine so that we can have the pleasure or satisfaction that comes from completing certain task. However there are substances that regulate this process and circumvents its natural ability to maintain a homeostatic physiology that is consistent with normal human responses.

When people become addicted to substances, their primary motivation and reward is to obtain that drug, and they will exhibit behaviors and all manners to obtain that drug, followed by impulsivity and compulsivity. Drug use becomes chronic in relations to trauma that are compounded and poorly resolved. Shortly after, in the recreational phase of drug use, the abuser will modulate stressful responses, situational dysfunction, and other forms of emotional disarray with the substance. This substance will then in turn cause and treat depression, so it's a cyclical effect that's very hard to come out of.

I usually encourage my patients to embrace a holistic approach with good nutrition therapy and family support if any or acquire a social network or join other support groups are offered by most churches or religious organizations.

Childhood trauma is a major component of substance abuse, and I highly enforce my bias towards people going into the field of psychology because they're trying to heal or understand some of their own psychological distress leading to their own dysfunction. I recommend that a person considering to study the field of psychology must ensure that they have dealt with all of their psychiatric distress to the point that they're able to treat another individual without being triggered from their past.

Substance abuse will often cause mood disorders, anxiety, and insomnia. Some patients also have quiet attention deficiencies resulting from their chronic substance abuse, and I do highly recommend psychotherapy and a good match of psychotropics for that particular patient. Patients should ensure that their therapist is able to build a therapeutic milieu in which trust is established, and they must be comfortable with their therapist; otherwise, the therapeutic nature of the session will be interrupted from the initial phase.

www.ingramcontent.com/pod-product-compliance
Lightning Source LLC
Chambersburg PA
CBHW031502210526
45463CB00003B/1039